Table of contents

Introduction

"Find your reason!"

Welcome to "No Excuse Fitness" – a short and simple guide to achieving optimal health and wellness, without any excuses holding you back. Are you tired of procrastinating on your fitness goals? Do you find yourself constantly coming up with excuses to avoid exercise and healthy habits? If so, this book is for you. In "No Excuse Fitness," we'll break down the barriers that have been holding you back from achieving your fitness goals, and provide you with practical strategies, tips, and techniques to overcome any excuse that may have been preventing you from living a healthy, active lifestyle.

Whether you are a beginner or an experienced fitness enthusiast, this book will empower you to take control of your health and fitness journey and unlock your full potential. Get ready to transform your mindset, overcome your excuses, and discover a new level of vitality and well-being through the power of "No Excuse Fitness." It's time to stop making excuses and start making progress toward the fit and healthy life you deserve. Are you ready to take the first step? Let's dive in!

<u>Chapter 1: Lifestyle and Habits: Building the Foundation for Health and Fitness Success</u>

"Fitness is not just a goal, it's a lifestyle. Make healthy choices, build positive habits, and transform your life!"

When it comes to achieving optimal health and fitness, it's not just about hitting the gym or following a strict diet. Your lifestyle and habits play a crucial role in your overall well-being. In this chapter, we'll delve into the importance of building a solid foundation of healthy lifestyle choices and habits that will support your fitness journey. By making positive changes in your daily routine, you can set yourself up for long-term success and create a sustainable healthy lifestyle that promotes health and fitness in all aspects of your life.

- Prioritize Sleep: Sleep is often overlooked but is a fundamental pillar of health and fitness. Quality sleep is essential for recovery, muscle growth, hormone regulation, and cognitive function. Aim for 7-9 hours of uninterrupted sleep each night and establish a consistent sleep schedule to optimize your body's natural sleep-wake cycle.

- Hydrate Properly: Staying hydrated is crucial for overall health and fitness. Water is essential for regulating body temperature, supporting digestion, and maintaining optimal performance during exercise. Make sure to drink plenty of water throughout the day, especially before and after workouts, and limit sugary beverages that can add unnecessary calories and negatively impact your health.

- Eat a Balanced Diet: A nutritious diet is the cornerstone of any fitness journey. Focus on consuming a variety of whole, nutrient-dense foods, including lean proteins, complex carbohydrates, healthy fats, and plenty of fruits and vegetables. Avoid processed foods, excessive added sugars, and unhealthy fats. Practice mindful eating to listen to your body's hunger and fullness cues.

- Move Regularly: Incorporate regular physical activity into your daily routine. Find activities you enjoy, such as walking, jogging, swimming, cycling, or dancing, and aim for at least 150 minutes of moderate-intensity aerobic activity per week. Incorporate strength training exercises to build muscle, improve bone density, and boost your metabolism.

- Manage Stress: Chronic stress can have detrimental effects on your health and fitness. Incorporate stress management techniques such as meditation, deep breathing, yoga, or other relaxation techniques into your routine. Prioritize self-care, set boundaries, and find healthy outlets to manage stress effectively.

- Limit Sedentary Behaviour: Minimize prolonged sitting and sedentary behaviour throughout your day. Incorporate regular movement breaks, take the stairs instead of the elevator, or stand while talking on the phone. Increasing your overall physical activity levels will contribute to improved health and fitness

- Surround Yourself with Support: Surrounding yourself with a positive support system can greatly impact your health and fitness journey. Seek out friends, family, or a fitness community that shares similar goals and values. Having someone to hold you accountable, provide motivation, and offer support can make a significant difference in your progress.
- Track Your Progress: Keep track of your fitness goals, achievements, and progress. Monitoring your workouts, nutrition, and other lifestyle habits can help you stay on track and make adjustments as needed. It also serves as a source of motivation and helps you celebrate your successes.
- Practice Consistency and Discipline: Building a healthy lifestyle and habits requires consistency and discipline. It's important to stay committed to your fitness journey, even when faced with challenges or setbacks. Embrace a growth mindset, be patient with yourself, and stay focused on your long-term health and fitness goals.

By incorporating these simple lifestyle changes and habits into your daily routine, you will create a solid foundation for your health and fitness journey. Remember, it's the small consistent changes over time that yield significant results. Building a healthy lifestyle and habits will support your overall health, boost your fitness levels, and set you up for long-term success on your fitness journey.

Chapter 2: Focus, Motivation, and Overcoming Excuses and Procrastination: Unlocking Your Inner Drive for Fitness Success

"Find a strong enough reason to overcome your weak excuses!"

When it comes to achieving your fitness goals, having focus and motivation are key factors that can make a significant difference in your success. Staying focused helps you maintain consistency, adhere to your workout routine, and make healthy choices, while motivation keeps you driven and determined to push through challenges and setbacks.

However, we all face challenges when it comes to staying focused, motivated, overcoming excuses, and avoiding procrastination. In this chapter, we will explore strategies and techniques to unlock your inner drive, overcome common excuses, and conquer procrastination to stay consistently focused and motivated on your fitness journey.

- Define Your "Why": Understanding your underlying motivation for pursuing fitness is crucial. Reflect on your reasons for wanting to improve your health and fitness. Is it to have more energy, reduce stress, feel confident, or set an example for loved ones? Identifying your "why" provides a compelling purpose that can fuel your motivation even when faced with challenges.

- Set SMART Goals: Establish specific, measurable, achievable, relevant, and time-bound (SMART) goals. Break your fitness journey into smaller, achievable targets that are aligned with your overall vision. This creates a clear roadmap that keeps you focused and motivated, as you track your progress and celebrate milestones along the way.

- Challenge Your Excuses: Excuses are one of the biggest barriers to staying motivated. Recognize and challenge the excuses that arise, such as lack of time, fatigue, or discomfort. Ask yourself if the excuse is valid or if it's just a roadblock that can be overcome with determination and prioritization. Reframe your mindset and shift from making excuses to finding solutions.

- Create a Plan: Develop a structured plan that outlines your fitness routine, schedule, and strategies to overcome potential obstacles. Having a plan in place helps you stay organized, sets your expectations, and minimizes room for procrastination. Create a routine that works for you and stick to it consistently.

- Find Your Fitness Passion: Engage in activities that you genuinely enjoy and that align with your interests and preferences. When you are passionate about your fitness routine, it becomes easier to stay motivated and committed. Experiment with different exercises, classes, or sports until you find what resonates with you.

- Enlist an Accountability Partner: Having someone to hold you accountable can be a powerful motivator. Find a workout buddy, a couch, or a mentor who can provide support, encouragement and help you stay on track. Share your goals and progress with them, and schedule regular check-ins to stay accountable.
- Use Positive Self-Talk and Visualize Success: Your inner dialogue can significantly impact your focus and motivation. Practice positive self-talk and replace negative thoughts or self-doubt with affirmations, encouragement, and motivation. Use the power of visualization to see yourself achieving your fitness goals. Create a mental picture of the future version of yourself, fit and healthy, and visualize yourself overcoming challenges and achieving success. Visualization can help reinforce your motivation and build belief in your capabilities.
- Manage Procrastination: Procrastination is a common roadblock to fitness success. Break tasks into smaller, manageable steps and tackle them one at a time. Avoid distractions, set deadlines, and practice self-discipline. Remember that taking action, even in small increments, is better than doing nothing at all.
- Reward Yourself: Celebrate your achievements along the way and reward yourself for your progress. Treat yourself to non-food rewards, such as a massage, a new workout outfit, or a day off. Acknowledging your hard work and progress boosts your motivation and reinforces positive habits.

- Stay Positive and Flexible: Maintaining a positive mindset and being adaptable to changes is key to overcoming obstacles and staying motivated. Embrace a growth mindset, be kind to yourself, and learn from setbacks. Be willing to adjust your plans as needed short term, and stay focused on your long-term goals.

- Embrace Progress, Not Perfection: Acknowledge and celebrate your progress, no matter how small. Avoid striving for perfection, as it can lead to discouragement and loss of motivation. Embrace the journey, focus on the improvements you're making, and be kind to yourself along the way. Remember that setbacks and challenges are part of the process, and use them as opportunities to learn and grow.

- Practice Mindfulness: Mindfulness is the practice of being present at the moment without judgment. Incorporating mindfulness techniques, such as deep breathing, meditation, or visualization can help you stay focused, reduce distractions and increase motivation during your workouts. It can also enhance your mind-muscle connection, allowing you to engage in your exercises more effectively.

By unlocking your inner drive, challenging excuses, and conquering procrastination, you can stay consistently motivated on your fitness journey. Remember that motivation is not always constant and may fluctuate over time. In the next chapter, we will look at some of the most common excuses to avoid exercise, fitness, or general overall health, and ways to overcome them.

MAKE YOUR REASONS STRONGER THAN YOUR EXCUSES

Chapter 3: Breaking Through the Top 5 Excuses and Barriers to Fitness Success

"Breakthrough, rise above and conquer your excuses. Smash your barriers and achieve your fitness success!"

When it comes to fitness, many people struggle with excuses and barriers that prevent them from taking action and achieving their goals. These excuses often serve as roadblocks that hinder progress and keep individuals from realizing their full fitness potential. In this chapter, we'll explore the top 5 excuses and barriers people often use to avoid fitness and discuss strategies to overcome them with motivation and determination.

- Lack of Time: One of the most common excuses people use to avoid fitness is a perceived lack of time. With busy schedules and competing priorities, it's easy to put exercise on the back burner. However, making time for fitness is essential for overall health and well-being.

Solution: Prioritize fitness as a non-negotiable part of your routine. Schedule regular workout sessions in your calendar, just like any other important appointment. Be realistic about your available time and find creative ways to fit in exercise, such as taking the stairs instead of the elevator, going for a walk on your lunch break, or incorporating short, intense workouts into your day (HIIT is a great way to accomplish this which we will cover later in the book). Remember that even a little bit of exercise is better than none. Consistency is key.

- Lack of Motivation: Another common barrier to fitness success is a lack of motivation. It's easy to lose steam and feel unmotivated, especially when facing challenges or setbacks along the way.

Solution: This goes back to finding your "why" as discussed in the previous chapter. Remind yourself of your underlying reasons and motivation for pursuing fitness. Reflect on the benefits of regular exercise, such as improved health, increased energy, reduced stress, and enhanced self-confidence. All of which you may have already noticed on your fitness journey, provided you've already started before the current lack of motivation to continue. Set specific and meaningful goals that inspire you to take action. Break your fitness journey into smaller manageable steps, and celebrate your progress to boost your motivation.

- Fear of Failure or Injury: Fear of failure or injury can hold people back from engaging in fitness activities. Worries about not being good enough or getting hurt can be powerful barriers that prevent individuals from even starting or pushing themselves to their full potential.

Solution: Reframe your mindset and view failure as an opportunity to learn and grow. There is a famous saying "We learn more from our mistakes and failures than from our success". This is true even when on a fitness journey, what works for one might not work for you, but you won't know unless you try. Embrace a growth mindset that focuses on progress rather than perfection. Start with activities that match your current fitness and capability levels and gradually progress. Seek guidance from a fitness professional to ensure proper form and technique to minimize the risk of injury. Remember that with proper guidance, preparation, and consistency, you can safely achieve your fitness goals.

- Lack of Support: A lack of support from family, friends, or peers can be discouraging and demotivating. Feeling alone or unsupported in your fitness journey can make it challenging to stay on track and maintain momentum.

Solution: Surround yourself with a supportive network that encourages and uplifts your fitness efforts. Share your goals and progress with loved ones, and ask for their support. Consider enlisting a workout buddy or finding a fitness community that shares similar interests and goals. Join fitness classes, sports teams, or online groups to connect with like-minded individuals who can provide motivation, inspiration, and accountability.

- Physical Limitations: Physical limitations, such as health conditions or injuries, can be significant barriers to fitness success. It's easy to use them as excuses to avoid exercise altogether.

Solution: Consult with your healthcare provider before starting or modifying an exercise program, especially if you have any health concerns or pre-existing conditions. Work with a fitness professional who can design a safe and effective exercise plan tailored to your specific needs and limitations. Be open to modifying your fitness routine based on your physical abilities and progress. Remember that exercise can often be adapted to accommodate different physical limitations, and staying active within your abilities is still beneficial for your health.

Conclusion:

Excuses and barriers can prevent us from achieving our fitness goals, but with determination, motivation, and a proactive mindset, we can overcome them. In this chapter, we explored the top 5 excuses and barriers people use to avoid fitness, including lack of time, motivation, the fear of failure or injury, a lack of support, and physical limitations. We also provided some insight and solutions to help overcome these barriers. Remember that taking small steps consistently, seeking support when needed, and maintaining a positive mindset can help you break through these excuses and barriers, and achieve success in your fitness journey. So, let's leave behind the excuses, overcome the barriers and commit ourselves to prioritizing our health and fitness for a better, more active, and fulfilling life!

NEVER GIVE UP.

STAY FOCUSED.

IT'S YOU VS YOU!

Chapter 4: The Power of Health and Fitness: Unlocking the Benefits of an Active Lifestyle

"Unlock the power within you through health and fitness. Embrace the strength, energy, and vitality that comes with living a fit and healthy lifestyle!"

In our fast-paced modern world, health, and fitness often take a backseat to busy schedules and competing priorities. However, incorporating regular exercise and leading an active lifestyle can have a profound positive impact on our physical, mental, and emotional well-being. In this chapter, we will explore the many benefits of prioritizing health and fitness in our lives.

- Improved physical health: Regular exercise has a myriad of benefits for our physical health. It helps to build and maintain strong muscles and bones, improve cardiovascular health, increase flexibility and mobility, and enhance our overall physical performance. Exercise also aids in weight management, reduces the risk of chronic diseases such as diabetes, hypertension, and obesity, and helps boost our immune system making us more resilient to illness.
- Increased energy and vitality: Engaging in regular physical activity can lead to increased energy levels and enhanced vitality. Exercise stimulates the production of endorphins, which are mood-boosting hormones that can help reduce stress, anxiety, and depression. It also improves our sleep

quality, helping us wake up feeling refreshed and rejuvenated, ready to tackle the day with renewed vigor.

- Enhanced mental health: Health and fitness have a profound impact on our mental well-being. Exercise has been shown to reduce symptoms of depression and anxiety, improve cognitive function and boost overall brain health. It can also increase our self-esteem, self-confidence, and self-efficacy, promoting a positive body image and a sense of accomplishment and empowerment.
- Increased productivity and focus: Leading an active lifestyle can improve our productivity and focus in all areas of our lives. Exercise increases blood flow to the brain, which enhances cognitive function, memory, and concentration. It also helps reduce stress, which can improve our ability to manage tasks, solve problems and make decisions effectively.
- Better quality of life: Prioritizing health and fitness can lead to a better overall quality of life. Regular exercise improves our physical capabilities, allowing us to participate in various activities and hobbies that we enjoy. It also promotes social connections and a sense of community as we engage in group fitness classes, sports teams, or outdoor activities with others. Leading an active lifestyle can also contribute to a longer lifespan, allowing us to enjoy more years of vitality and well-being.
- Increased confidence and self-esteem: Exercise and physical activity can greatly impact our self-confidence and self-esteem. As we challenge ourselves physically and achieve our fitness goals, we develop a sense of accomplishment and pride in our abilities. This increased confidence and self-

esteem can extend beyond the realm of fitness, positively affecting our personal and professional lives.

- Reduced stress and improved mental resilience: Exercise is a natural stress reliever that helps reduce the negative effects of stress on our bodies and minds. Regular physical activity can improve our ability to cope with stress, increase our mental resilience, and improve our emotional well-being. It provides an outlet for releasing tension and clearing our minds, allowing us to better manage the daily stressors of life.

Conclusion:

Health and fitness are powerful tools that can positively impact our physical, mental, and emotional well-being. Regular exercise and leading an active lifestyle offer a multitude of benefits, including improved physical health, increased energy and vitality, enhanced mental health, increased productivity and focus, better quality of life, increased confidence and self-esteem, and reduced stress. By prioritizing health and fitness in our lives, we can unlock these benefits and experience a more fulfilling, healthy, and happy life. So, let's embrace the power of health and fitness and make it a priority in our daily lives!

Chapter 5: Lifestyle Habits

"A few simple changes to your lifestyle can make a big impact!"

While adjusting current lifestyle habits can be difficult, especially ones that you've been doing for years but aren't helping your health or fitness, making small changes over time can make a big difference. I understand that designing a weekly lifestyle habit that fits into a normal 9-hour working day, 5 days a week can be challenging, but with some planning and dedication it's achievable. So here are some suggested weekly lifestyle habits that can aid in improving your health and fitness.

Monday to Friday:

- Morning exercise routine: Start your day with a short but effective exercise routine to kickstart your metabolism and energize your body. You can do a quick workout at home, such as bodyweight exercises, yoga, or a short cardio session. Aim for at least 20-30 minutes to get your heart rate up and boost your mood for the day. (A suggested morning workout will be at the end of this chapter).
- Healthy packed lunch: Plan and prepare healthy packed lunches for work. Aim for balanced meals that include lean protein, whole grains, plenty of vegetables, and healthy fats. Avoid processed foods, sugary snacks, and excessive caffeine. Bringing your own lunch allows you to have

control over the quality and quantity of food you consume, helping you make healthier choices and avoid temptations.

- Active breaks: Make a conscious effort to take active breaks during your workday. Instead of sitting at your desk for prolonged periods, take short breaks to stand, stretch or go for a short walk. You can also incorporate some light exercises or stretches, such as squats, lunges, or desk yoga to keep your muscles engaged and improve circulation.

- Prioritize sleep: Getting enough quality sleep is crucial for overall health and fitness. Aim for 7-9 hours of sleep each night to allow your body to repair and recover from the day's activities. Establish a consistent sleep schedule and create a relaxing bedtime routine to help you wind down and prepare for restorative sleep.

- Mindful eating: Practice mindful eating by paying attention to your hunger and fullness cues, eating slowly, and avoiding distractions such as screens while eating. Listen to your body's signal and eat mindfully, savour each bite, and enjoy your meals without rushing. This can help prevent overeating and promote better digestion.

Weekend:

- Outdoor activities: Utilize your weekends to engage in outdoor activities that you enjoy such as hiking, biking, swimming, or playing sports. Outdoor activities not only provide physical exercise but also offer mental and emotional benefits from being in nature and getting fresh air.

- Meal prep: Take some time on the weekends to meal prep for the upcoming week. Plan and prepare healthy meals in advance so you have nutritious options readily available during busy workdays. This can help you stay on track with your healthy eating goals and avoid last-minute unhealthy food choices. (A few suggested meal prep ideas will be in the next chapter).

- Rest and recovery: Allow yourself to rest and recover during the weekends to avoid burnout and support your body's healing process. Engage in activities that help you relax and de-stress, such as meditation, yoga, or taking a bath. Prioritize self-care and make time for activities that help you recharge physically and mentally.

Remember, consistency is key when it comes to establishing healthy lifestyle habits. It's important to find a routine that works for you and fits into your schedule and to make gradual changes that are sustainable in the long run. With commitment and dedication, you can create a weekly lifestyle habit that aids in your health and fitness goals, even with a busy 9-hour working day.

Morning workout

"Rise and shine, energize and thrive! Fuel your day with a morning workout to kickstart your body and soul!"

An ideal morning workout should be efficient and effective, providing a burst of energy to kickstart your day. Here's a suggested 20-minute morning workout routine that can help you start your day on the right foot.

Warm-up (3 minutes):

- Jumping jacks – 1 minute.
- Dynamic stretching (E.g., arm circles, leg swings, hip circles) – 1 minute
- Bodyweight exercises (E.g., squats, lunges, push up's) 1 minute

Cardiovascular Exercise (7 minutes):

- High knees – 1 minute
- Burpees – 1 minute
- Jump rope (real or imaginary) – 2 minutes
- Mountain climbers – 1 minute
- Fast-paced walk or jog in place – 2 minutes

Strength training (7 minutes):

- Bodyweight squats – 1 minute
- Push-ups (on knees or toes) – 1 minute
- Plank – 1 minute
- Triceps dips (using chair or bench) – 1 minute
- Russian twists (with or without weight) – 2 minutes

Cool-down and stretching (3 minutes):

- Slow walking or marching in place – 1 minute
- Static stretching (E.g., hamstring stretch. chest stretch, quad stretch) – 2 minutes

Remember to always listen to your body and modify exercises or intensity levels as needed. If you're new to exercise or have any health concerns, it's best to consult with a healthcare professional before starting a new workout routine.

In addition to the physical benefits, a morning workout can also help improve mood, increase productivity, and set a positive tone for the rest of your day. Remember to stay hydrated throughout your workout and follow it up with a nutritious breakfast to refuel your body for the day ahead. Make sure to also cool down and stretch to promote flexibility and prevent muscle soreness.

Starting your day with a 20-minute workout can be a powerful way to prioritize your health and fitness and set the tone for a productive and energizes day ahead.

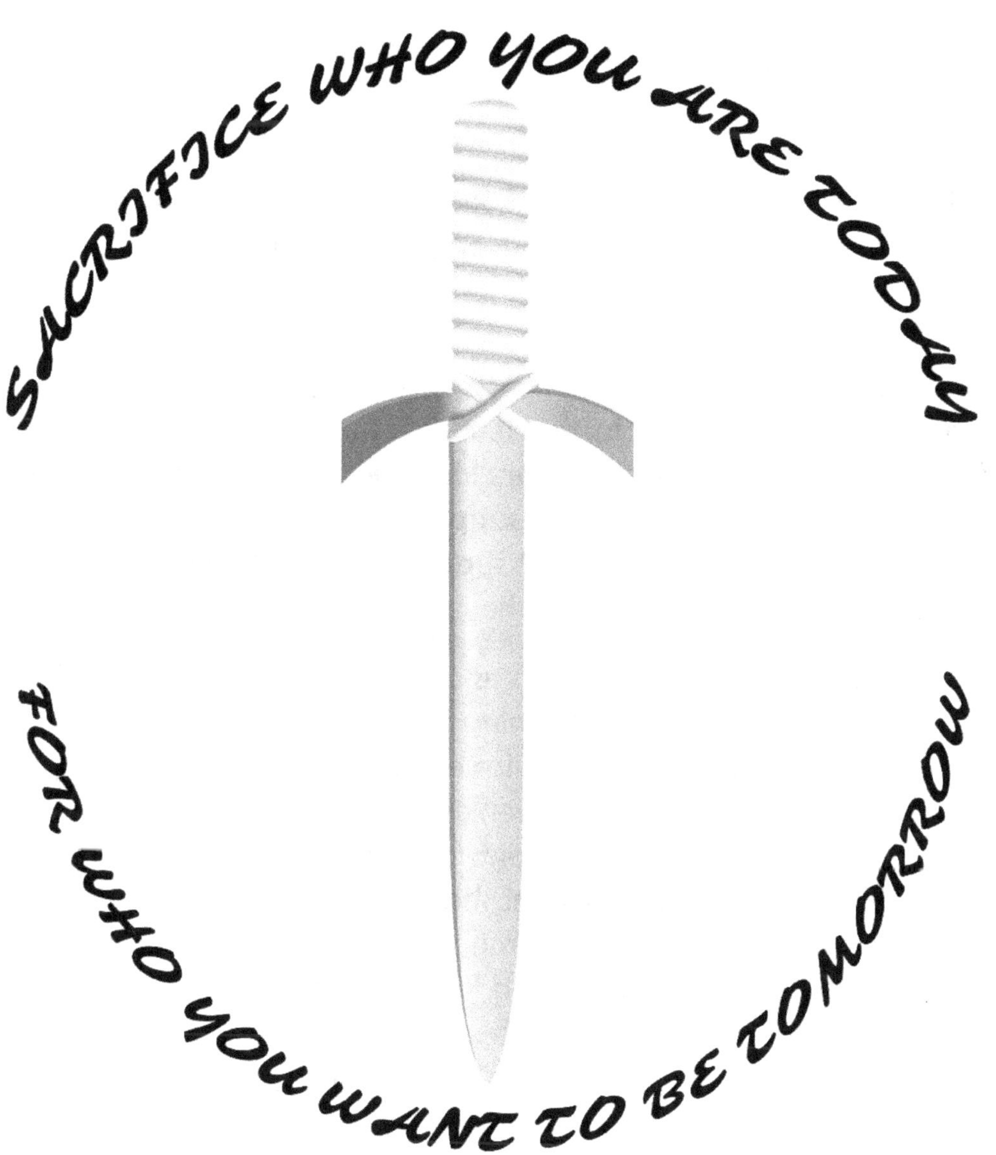

SACRIFICE WHO YOU ARE TODAY
FOR WHO YOU WANT TO BE TOMORROW

Chapter 6: Food and Supplements

"Never underestimate the power of supplements or the benefits of eating properly balanced meals."

When it comes to health and fitness, a well-balanced diet that includes a variety of whole, nutrient-rich foods should be the foundation of your nutrition plan. However, certain supplements can complement your diet and support your health and fitness goals. Here are some of the best supplements for health and fitness, along with reasons why they can be beneficial:

- Protein powder: Protein is essential for muscle building, repair, and recovery, making it an important nutrient for those who engage in regular exercise or strength training. Protein powders are convenient and versatile, making them a popular supplement for fitness enthusiasts. They can be used as a post-workout shake to support muscle recovery or as a snack or meal replacement to help meet protein requirements. Look for a high-quality protein powder that contains all the essential amino acids and minimal added sugars or artificial ingredients.

- Omega-3 fatty acids: Omega-3 fatty acids are essential fats that have been shown to have numerous health benefits, including reducing inflammation, supporting heart health, and improving brain function. They are commonly found in fatty fish like salmon, but can also be taken as a supplement in the form of fish oil or algae-based supplements. Omega-3 fatty acids are particularly beneficial for those who engage in intense exercise or endurance training as they can help reduce inflammation and promote recovery.

- Vitamin D: vitamin D is an important nutrient that plays a role in bone health, immune function, and muscle function. It is synthesized in the skin when exposed to sunlight, but many people may have inadequate levels, especially during winter months or for those with limited sun exposure. Vitamin D supplements can benefit those with low levels of sun exposure, who live in northern latitudes or have a higher risk of vitamin D deficiency. However, it's important to talk to your healthcare provider to determine the appropriate dosage for your individual needs. When looking for vitamin D supplements try and find one that is D3 and K2 in one as the vitamin K2 helps the body absorb and utilize the vitamin D more efficiently.
- Creatine: Creatine is a naturally occurring compound found in small amounts in meat and fish. It is effective in improving strength, power, and performance in high-intensity, short-duration activities such as weightlifting or sprinting. Creatine supplements can help increase muscle creatine levels, which help lead to improved exercise performance and muscle gains. It's important to note that creatine may not be suitable for everyone and should be used under the guidance of a healthcare professional, especially if you have any underlying health conditions.
- Multivitamin/Multimineral supplements: A well-balanced diet should provide all the essential vitamins and minerals

your body needs, but some individuals may have nutrient gaps due to dietary restrictions, limited food choices, or other factors. A high-quality multivitamin/multimineral supplement can help fill these nutrient gaps and support overall health and well-being. Look for a reputable brand that provides the recommended daily allowance (RDA) for a wide range of vitamins and minerals, and avoid mega-doses or excessive supplementation, as this can have potential risks.

It's important to note that supplements should not be viewed as a substitute for a healthy diet and lifestyle. They are meant to complement a well-balanced diet and exercise routine and should be used under the guidance of a healthcare professional to ensure safety and efficacy. Always consult your healthcare provider before starting any new supplement regimen, especially if you have any underlying health conditions or are taking long-term medications. Additionally, choosing high-quality supplements from reputable sources is crucial to ensure their safety and effectiveness.

As discussed in the previous chapter about organizing your lifestyle habits, meal prepping is a great way to save time during the days you have work or have other commitments that leave you short on time. It is also a fantastic way to ensure you have nutritious meals ready after intense physical training. Below are five meal prep ideas suited for post-workout recovery and can be prepared days in advance:

1. Grilled Chicken with Quinoa and Roasted Vegetables

- Grill chicken breasts in advance and season with your favourite herbs and spices.
- Cook quinoa according to package instructions and refrigerate.
- Chop up a variety of vegetables (such as bell peppers, broccoli, and carrots), toss with olive oil, salt, and pepper, and roast in the oven.
- Portion the grilled chicken, quinoa, and roasted vegetables into meal prep containers for a balance and protein-rich post-workout meal.

2. Veggie Stir-fry with Brown rice:
   - Cook brown rice in advance and refrigerate.
   - Chop up a mix of colourful vegetables (such as bell peppers, mushrooms, snap peas, and carrots).
   - Heat a non-stick skillet with a little bit of oil and stir-fry the veggies until crisp-tender.
   - Toss the stir-fried veggies with your favourite stir-fry sauce (such as teriyaki or soy sauce) and let it cool before portioning out with the brown rice in meal prep containers.

3. Lentil and Vegetable Curry with Quinoa:
   - Cook lentils in advance and refrigerate.
   - Chop up an array of vegetables (such as sweet potatoes, cauliflower, and spinach).
   - In a large pot, sauté onions, garlic, and ginger with curry powder or paste.
   - Add in the chopped vegetables, cooked lentils, and coconut milk, and let it simmer until the vegetable are tender.

- Cook quinoa separately and portion out the lentil and vegetable curry with quinoa in meal prep containers for a wholesome and flavourful post-workout meal

4. Greek salad with Grilled Chicken
   - Grill chicken breasts in advance and refrigerate.
   - Prepare a Greek salad with a mix of fresh vegetables and fruits (such as tomatoes, cucumbers, red onions, and olives) and feta cheese.
   - Make a simple vinaigrette with olive oil, lemon juice, garlic, and dried oregano.
   - Portion out the Greek salad into meal prep containers and top with sliced grilled chicken for a refreshing and protein-packed post-workout meal.

5. Black Bean and Veggie burrito bowl:
   - Cook black beans in advance and refrigerate.
   - Chop up an assortment of vegetables (such as bell peppers, onions, corn, and tomatoes).
   - Sauté the veggies in a pan with some oil and season with cumin, chili powder, and paprika for a Mexican-inspired flavour.
   - Cook brown rice separately and portion out the black beans, sauteed veggies, and brown rice into meal prep containers.
   - Top with avocado slices, salsa, and Greek yogurt for a delicious and satisfying post-workout burrito bowl.

Remember to store your meal prep containers in the refrigerator and reheat them as needed. These meal prep ideas are versatile and can be customized based on your dietary preferences and fitness goals. They provide a good balance of carbohydrates, protein, and healthy fats to support muscle recovery and replenish energy after intense physical training. Happy meal prepping and enjoy your delicious and nutritious post-workout meals.

More meal ideas for inspiration

Below are some more meal ideas that will hopefully inspire you to try and shake up the normal routine and move away from processed/fast food. Below we'll go over a complete 7-day meal plan that is ideal for building muscle and strength (strength training-focused workouts). Hopefully, it will help you build your meal plan, should there be anything not to your fancy feel free to switch it up.

7-day meal plan:

Day 1:

Breakfast: Veggie omelette made with eggs, spinach, bell peppers, and cheese. Served with whole-grain toast.

Snack: Greek yogurt with mixed berries and a handful of nuts.

Lunch: Grilled chicken breast with roasted vegetables (such as broccoli, carrots, and Brussels sprouts) and quinoa.

Snack: Apple slice with almond butter.

Dinner: Baked salmon with steamed asparagus and sweet potato.

Day 2:

Breakfast: Overnight oats made with rolled oats, milk, Greek yogurt, chia seeds, and sliced bananas.

Snack Cottage cheese with diced pineapple.

Lunch: Lean beef stir-fry with mixed vegetables (such as bell peppers, mushrooms, and bok choy) and brown rice.

Snack: Baby carrots with hummus

Dinner: Grilled turkey breast with roasted green beans and mashed cauliflower.

Day 3:

Breakfast: Protein smoothie made with whey protein powder, frozen berries, spinach, and almond milk.

Snack: Hard-boiled eggs with cherry tomatoes.

Lunch: Black bean and vegetable chilli with avocado and quinoa.

Snack: Greek yogurt with honey and mixed nuts.

Dinner: Grilled shrimp with roasted zucchini and quinoa.

Day 4:

Breakfast: Whole grain pancakes with banana and walnuts, topped with Greek yogurt and drizzled with maple syrup.

Snack: Fresh fruit salad.

Lunch: Grilled chicken breast with steamed broccoli and brown rice.

Snack: Cottage cheese with diced mango.

Dinner: Baked tofu with roasted vegetables (such as cauliflower, carrots, and bell peppers) and quinoa.

Day 5:

Breakfast: Veggie and cheese omelette made with eggs, tomatoes, spinach, and feta cheese. Served with whole-grain toast.

Snack: Mixed nuts with dried fruit.

Lunch: Lentil and vegetable stew with whole grain bread.

Snack: Greek yogurt with mixed berries.

Dinner: Grilled steak with roasted asparagus and sweet potato.

Day 6:

Breakfast: Protein-packed breakfast burrito with eggs, black beans, bell peppers, and avocado wrapped in a whole-grain tortilla.

Snack: Apple slices with peanut butter.

Lunch: Grilled fish (such as cod or tilapia) with roasted vegetables and quinoa.

Snack: cottage cheese with diced peaches.

Dinner: Baked chicken thighs with roasted Brussels sprouts and mashed sweet potato.

Day 7:

Breakfast: Quinoa porridge with almond milk, dried fruit, and chopped nuts.

Snack: Greek yogurt with honey and fresh fruit.

Lunch: Veggie burger with whole grain bun, topped with lettuce, tomato, and avocado. Served with roasted vegetables.

Snack: Hard-boiled eggs with baby carrots.

Dinner: Grilled salmon with roasted mixed vegetables and brown rice.

CHECKLIST

- FIND REASON
- PACK BAG
- HIT THE GYM
- IGNORE NEGITIVITY

Chapter 7: Workouts

"Dedication is the key to success; Rome wasn't built in a day."

In this chapter, we get onto the good stuff, workout ideas. First up we will cover a 7-day strength and hypertrophy workout suggestion aimed at building strength while also promoting muscle growth to improve size and definition. Then we'll have a HIIT program designed to burn calories and get the weight falling off. After that, we'll get onto calisthenics and bodyweight training aimed at maximizing muscle definition and providing you with a way to workout without needing to get to a gym. Remember that no matter what type of workout you plan to do always ensure to warm up and cool down correctly.

Strength and hypertrophy

Day 1: Chest and Triceps

1. Bench Press: 4 sets of 8-10 reps
2. Incline dumbbell bench press: 3 sets of 10-12 reps
3. Chest flyers: 3 sets of 10-12 reps
4. Tricep dips: 3 sets of 12-15 reps
5. Tricep pushdowns: 3 sets of 12-15 reps
6. Close-grip bench press: 3 sets of 8-10 reps

Day 2: Back and Biceps

1. Deadlifts: 4 sets of 6-8 reps

2. Pull-ups or Chin-ups: 3 sets of max reps (use bands or assistance if needed)
3. Bent over rows: 3 sets of 10-12 reps
4. Lat pulldowns: 3 sets of 10-12 reps
5. Bicep curls: 3 sets of 10-12 reps
6. Hammer curls: 3 sets of 10-12 reps

Day 3: Rest Day or active recovery (e.g. light walking, stretching, and yoga)

Day 4: Legs

1. Squats: 4 sets of 8-10 reps
2. Romanian deadlifts: 3 sets of 10-12 reps
3. Leg press: 3 sets of 10-12 reps
4. Lunges: 3 sets of 10-12 reps per leg
5. Leg curls: 3 sets of 10-12 reps
6. Calf raises: 3 sets of 15-20 reps

Day 5: Shoulders and Abs

1. Shoulder press: 4 sets of 8-10 reps
2. Lateral raises: 3 sets of 10-12 reps
3. Upright rows: 3 sets of 10-12 reps
4. Front raises: 3 sets of 10-12 reps
5. Plank: 3 sets of 30-60 seconds
6. Russian twists: 3 sets of 20 reps (10 reps per side)
7. Hanging leg/knee raises: 3 sets of 10-15 reps

Day 6: Arms

1. Barbell curls: 3 sets of 10-12 reps
2. Preacher curls: 3 sets of 10-12 reps
3. Concentration curls: 3 sets of 10-12 reps per arm

4. Skull crushers: 3 sets of 10-12 reps
5. Overhead tricep extension: 3 sets of 10-12 reps
6. Close grip bench press: 3 sets of 8-10 reps

Day 7: Rest Day or Active Recovery.

Rest in-between sets for 45-90 seconds. To maximize hypertrophy, you want to keep your reps in the 8-15 range and weights at about 60-70% of your one rep max however, this is a guideline. Remember to adjust the weights, sets, and reps to your fitness level, especially if just starting on a weight training program, and always prioritize proper form and safety. Allow for adequate rest days and listen to your body. Proper nutrition and hydration are also crucial for muscle hypertrophy, so make sure to fuel your body with nutritious foods and stay hydrated throughout your training program. Consult with a qualified fitness professional before starting any new exercise program, especially if you have any pre-existing health conditions or concerns.

HIIT (High-Intensity Interval Training)

In today's fast-paced world, finding efficient and effective workout routines that fit into busy schedules is a top priority for many fitness enthusiasts. High-intensity Interval Training (HIIT) has gained popularity as a time-efficient and highly effective workout method that combines short bursts of intense exercise with brief recovery periods. This chapter will explore the benefits, principles, and guidelines of HIIT, as well as provide examples of HIIT workouts that can be incorporated into your fitness routine.

Benefits of HIIT:

HIIT offers a variety of benefits that make it an attractive option for those looking to maximize their workout results in a limited amount of time. Some of the key benefits of HIIT include:

1. Time efficiency: HIIT workouts typically last for 20-30 minutes, making them a time-efficient option for busy individuals who may not have hours to spend in the gym.
2. Increased calorie burns: HIIT workouts are known for their ability to boost calorie burn during and after the workout. The intense bursts of exercise increase your heart rate and metabolic rate, resulting in a higher calorie burn even after you've finished your workout.
3. Improved cardiovascular fitness: HIIT involves high-intensity exercises that challenge your cardiovascular system, leading to improved cardiovascular endurance and performance.
4. Muscle building and strength development: HIIT workouts often incorporate strength training exercises, which can help build lean muscle mass, improve strength, and enhance overall body composition.
5. Flexibility and adaptability: HIIT workouts can be adapted to suit different fitness levels, making them accessible to individuals of varying fitness levels from beginners to advanced exercisers.

Principles of HIIT:

HIIT follows specific principles that define its structure and effectiveness. Some key principles of HIIT include:

1. Intensity: HIIT workouts are characterized by short bursts of high-intensity exercise, where you push yourself to work at or near your maximum effort level during intense intervals.
2. Interval duration: HIIT involves alternating periods of high-intensity exercise with short recovery periods. The duration of intervals can vary, but typically, the intense intervals last for 20-60 seconds, followed by recovery periods of 10-60 seconds.
3. Varied exercises: HIIT workouts can incorporate a wide variety of exercises, including cardiovascular exercises like running, cycling, or jumping rope, as well as bodyweight exercises, resistance training, and more.
4. Progressive overload: Similar to other forms of exercise, progressive overload is important in HIIT to continue challenging your body and promoting continuous improvement. This can be achieved by increasing the intensity, duration, or complexity of the exercises over time.

Guidelines for HIIT:

To get the most out of your HIIT workouts, it's important to follow some guidelines to ensure safety and effectiveness. Here are some general guidelines for incorporating HIIT into your fitness routine:

1. Warm-up and cool-down: Always start your HIIT workout with a warm-up to prepare your body for the intense exercise and end with a cool-down to help your body transition back to a resting state.
2. Start at your fitness level: HIIT can be intense, so it's important to start at a level that matches your fitness capabilities. Beginners may need to start with shorter

intervals or lower intensity, while more advanced exercisers can push themselves to work at higher intensity levels.

3. Listen to your body: Pay attention to your body's signals and adjust the intensity or duration of the intervals as needed. It's important to avoid pushing yourself to the point of exhaustion or risking injury.

4. Focus on proper form: Maintaining proper form during the exercises is essential for safety and effectiveness. Make sure you are performing the exercises with proper technique and alignment to prevent injury and maximize the benefits of HIIT.

5. Plan for rest and recovery: HIIT workouts are intense and can put a lot of stress on your muscles and cardiovascular system. It's crucial to allow your body enough time to recover between HIIT sessions to prevent overtraining and promote optimal performance.

6. Modify as needed: HIIT workouts can be adapted to suit different fitness levels, preferences, and goals. You can modify the intensity, duration, or exercises to fit your specific needs and make HIIT workouts a sustainable part of your fitness routine.

Examples of HIIT workouts:

1. Cardio HIIT: Perform 30 seconds of high-intensity exercises such as burpees, mountain climbers, or high knees, followed by 30 seconds of active rest like walking or jogging. Repeat for 10-15 rounds.

2. Bodyweight HIIT: Perform 45 seconds of bodyweight exercises such as squats, push-ups, lunges, or plank, followed by 15 seconds of rest. Repeat for 5-7 rounds.

3. Tabata HIIT: Perform 20 seconds of all-out effort on one exercise, followed by 10 seconds of rest. Repeat for 8 rounds, totaling 4 minutes. You can choose exercises like jump squats, sprints, or kettlebell swings.
4. Strength HIIT: Perform a circuit of strength training exercises such as dumbbell squats, kettlebell swings, push presses, and rows for 45 seconds each, followed by 15 seconds of rest. Repeat for 3-4 rounds.
5. Pyramid HIIT: Perform a series of exercises in a pyramid format, starting with 10 seconds of work, followed by 10 seconds of rest. Then increase the work time to 20 seconds, followed by 10 seconds of rest, and continue to increase until you reach the peak of the pyramid, and then decrease back down. You can choose exercises like jumping jacks, burpees, or high knees.

A full HIIT workout example:

Warm-up (5 minutes):

1. Jumping jacks: 60 seconds
2. Bodyweight squats: 60 seconds
3. Mountain climbers: 60 seconds
4. Dynamic stretching (e.g., arm circles, leg swings): 60 seconds

HIIT circuit (15 minutes): Perform each exercise for 40 seconds, followed by a 20 seconds' rest. Repeat the circuit for 3 rounds.

1. Burpees
2. High knees
3. Jumping lunges
4. Push-ups
5. Plank jacks

6. Bicycle crunches
7. Box jumps or Step-ups
8. Russian Twists

Cool-down (5 minutes):

1. Walking or jogging in place: 60 seconds
2. Static stretching (e.g., hamstring stretch, shoulder stretch): 60 seconds per muscle group
3. Deep breathing: 60 seconds

High-Intensity Interval Training (HIIT) is a popular effective workout method that can help you achieve your fitness goals in a time-efficient manner. By incorporating short bursts of high-intensity exercise with brief recovery periods. HIIT can improve cardiovascular fitness, build lean muscle mass, and boost calorie burn. Following the principles and guidelines of HIIT, and modifying as needed can help you safely and effectively incorporate HIIT into your fitness routine. Experiment with different exercises, durations, and intensities to find what works best for you and make HIIT a fun and challenging part of your fitness journey.

Calisthenics

Calisthenics, also known as bodyweight training, is a form of exercise that utilizes the resistance of your body weight to build strength, flexibility, and endurance. Calisthenics exercises can be performed using little to no equipment, making them accessible and versatile for people of all fitness levels. In the subchapters, we will delve into the world of calisthenics and explore its benefits, key principles, and how to incorporate it into your fitness routine.

<u>Benefits of calisthenics</u>

Calisthenics offers a wide range of benefits that can enhance your physical fitness and overall well-being. Some of the key benefits of calisthenics include:

- Increased strength: Calisthenics exercises target multiple muscle groups, helping you build functional strength that can be applied to real-life movements and activities.
- Improved flexibility: Many calisthenics exercises require flexibility and mobility, helping you improve your range of motion and overall flexibility.
- Enhanced endurance: Calisthenics workouts often involve high-rep sets and circuits, which can improve your cardiovascular endurance and muscular endurance over time.
- Versatility: Calisthenics exercises can be adapted to different fitness levels, making them suitable for beginners, intermediate, and advanced individuals.
- Convenience: Calisthenics can be performed anywhere, anytime, without the need for expensive equipment or a gym membership, making it a convenient option for those with busy schedules or limited access to a gym.
- Functional fitness: Calisthenics exercises mimic natural human movements, helping you develop functional fitness

that can improve your performance in daily activities and sports.

- Body awareness: Calisthenics requires body control, balance, and coordination, helping you develop better body awareness and proprioception.

<u>Key principles of calisthenics</u>

Calisthenics is based on a few key principles that are essential to its effectiveness:

- Progressive overload: Just like other forms of strength training, progressive overload is crucial in calisthenics. You need to continually challenge your muscles by increasing the resistance, changing the leverage, or progressing to more advanced exercises to keep making gains in strength and muscle development.
- Proper technique: Proper technique is important in calisthenics to ensure effective and safe execution of exercises. Focus on using proper form and technique for each exercise to maximize its benefits and minimize the risk of injury
- Full body training: Calisthenics exercises often engage multiple muscle groups simultaneously, providing a full-body workout. It's important to include exercises that target all major muscle groups, including upper body, lower body, core, and back, for a well-rounded and balanced workout.
- Mobility and flexibility: Calisthenics requires good mobility and flexibility for proper execution of exercises. Incorporating exercises that improve your flexibility and

mobility, such as stretching and mobility drills, can help you perform calisthenics movements with better form and effectiveness.

- Rest and recovery: Rest and recovery are crucial for muscle growth and overall performance. It's important to allow your muscles to recover and repair by scheduling rest days and avoiding overtraining, especially when engaging in intense calisthenics workouts.

Incorporating calisthenics into your fitness routine

Here are some tips on how to incorporate calisthenics into your fitness routine:

- Start with the basics: If you're new to calisthenics, start with the basic exercises that match your fitness level. Master the foundational exercises, such as push-ups, pull-ups, squats, dips, and planks, before progressing to more advanced variations.

- Progress gradually: Calisthenics allow for progressive overload, so aim to gradually increase the difficulty of your exercises over time. This can be achieved by increasing the number of repetitions, changing the leverage, or progressing to more challenging variations of the exercises.

- Create a balanced routine: A well-rounded calisthenics routine should include exercises that target all major muscle groups, including the chest, back, shoulders, arms, legs, and core. Aim to create a balanced routine that covers all areas of your body for a comprehensive workout.

- Incorporate mobility and flexibility exercises: Flexibility and mobility are important for effective calisthenics training.

Include exercises that improve your flexibility and mobility, such as stretching, mobility drills, and yoga, to enhance your overall performance and reduce the risk of injury.

- Schedule rest days: Rest and recovery are crucial for muscle growth and overall performance. Make sure to schedule rest days in your calisthenics routine to allow your muscles to recover and repair. Overtraining can lead to decreased performance and increased risk of injury, so listen to your body and prioritize rest.
- Track your progress: Keep track of your progress to monitor your improvements and stay motivated. Keep a record of your exercise routines, the number of repetitions, and the level of difficulty to see how far you've come and set goals for yourself.
- Pay attention to nutrition: As with all forms of training and exercise proper nutrition is essential for supporting your calisthenics workouts and optimizing your performance. Make sure to fuel your body with balanced meals that provide enough protein, carbohydrates, and healthy fats to support muscle growth, recovery, and overall health.

<u>Sample calisthenics workout</u>

Here's a sample 1-hour calisthenics workout routine that you can incorporate into your fitness routine, further on is a 5-day calisthenics workout plan for your inspiration:

Warm Up (5-10 minutes):

- Dynamic stretching (arm circles, leg swings, etc.)
- Mobility drills (shoulder rolls, hip circles, etc.)

Main workout (45-50 minutes):

- Pull-ups (3 sets of 8-10 reps)
- Push-ups (3 sets of 12-15 reps)
- Dips (3 sets of 10-12 reps)
- Squats (3 sets of 15-20 reps)
- Plank (3 sets of 30-60 secs)
- Lunges (3 sets of 10-12 reps per leg)
- Inverted rows (3 sets of 10-12 reps)
- Hanging leg raises (3 sets of 10-12 reps)

Cool-down (5-10 minutes):

- Static stretching (hamstring stretch. chest stretch, etc.)
- Deep breathing and relaxation exercises

Note: This is just a sample routine, and the number of sets, reps, and exercises can be adjusted to your fitness level and goals. It's important to consult with a qualified fitness professional before starting any new exercise routine, especially if you have any health concerns or medical conditions.

Conclusion

Calisthenics is a versatile and effective form of exercise that can help you build strength, flexibility, and endurance using your body weight. By incorporating calisthenics into your fitness routine, you can achieve a well-rounded workout that targets all major muscle groups and improves your overall physical fitness. Remember to start with the basics, progress gradually, prioritize rest and recovery, and pay attention to proper nutrition to optimize your calisthenics training. With consistency and dedication, you can master the art of calisthenics and dedication, you can master of calisthenics and unleash the full potential of your body.

<u>5-day calisthenics training</u>

Day 1: upper body

Warm-up:

- Jumping jacks: 3 sets of seconds
- Arm circles: 3 sets of 10 seconds (forward and backward)
- Push up to downward dog stretch: 3 sets of 5 reps

Workout:

- Pull-ups (or chin-ups): 3 sets of max reps (use bands or assistance if needed)
- Push-ups: 3 sets of 15-20 reps
- Dips (on parallel bars or using a sturdy chair): 3 sets of 10-15 reps
- Inverted rows (using a bar or TRX straps): 3 sets of 10-15 reps
- Diamond push-ups: 3 sets of 10-15 reps
- Plank: 3 sets of 30-60 seconds

Day 2: Lower body

Warm-up:

- Jumping jacks: 3 sets of 30 seconds
- Leg swings (forward and sideways): 3 sets of 10 reps per leg
- Bodyweight squats: 3 sets of 15 reps

Workout:

- Pistol squats (or assisted pistol squats): 3 sets of 8-10 reps per leg
- Bulgarian split squats: 3 sets of 10-12 reps per leg
- Glute bridges: 3 sets of 15-20 reps
- Step-ups (on a box or bench): 3 sets of 10-12 reps per leg
- Calf raises: 3 sets of 15-20 reps
- Hanging knee raises: 3 sets of 10-15 reps

Day 3: Rest Day or active recovery (E.g. light walking, stretching, yoga)

Day 4: Full body

Warm-up:

- Jumping jacks: 3 sets of seconds
- Arm circles: 3 sets of 10 seconds (forward and backward)
- Bodyweight squats: 3 sets of 15 reps

Workout:

- Handstand practice (against a wall or freestanding): 3 sets of 30-60 seconds
- Pull-ups (or chin-ups): 3 sets of max reps (use bands or assistance if needed)
- Push-ups: 3 sets of 15-20 reps
- Bodyweight rows (using a bar or TRX straps): 3 sets of 10-15 reps
- Dips (on parallel bars or using a sturdy chair): 3 sets of 10-15 reps

- Bodyweight lunges: 3 sets of 10-12 reps per leg

Day 5: Core and cardio

Warm-up:

- Jumping jacks: 3 sets of 30 seconds
- Leg swings (forward and sideways): 3 sets of 10 reps per leg
- Plank: 3 sets of 30-60 seconds

Workout:

- Hanging leg raises: 3 sets of 10-15 reps
- Russian twists: 3 sets of 20 reps (10 reps per side)
- Bicycle crunches: 3 sets of 20 reps (10 reps per side)
- Flutter kicks: 3 sets of 30 seconds
- High knees: 3 sets of 30 seconds
- Burpees: 3 sets of 10-12 reps

Remember to adjust the reps and sets to your fitness level, and always prioritize proper form and safety. Allow rest between sets of 30-90 seconds, and always warm up and cool down before and after each workout.

As a bonus to this chapter to help you build your workout routine here are what many consider the top 5 exercises for each of the major muscle groups.

Chest:
- Barbell bench press
- Dumbbell bench press
- Push-ups

* Chest flyes
* Incline bench press

Back:
* Pull-ups
* Deadlifts
* Bent-over rows
* Lat pull-downs
* T-bar rows

Legs:
* Squats
* Deadlifts
* Lunges
* Leg press
* Bulgarian split squats

Shoulders:
* Overhead press (barbell or dumbbell)
* Lateral raises
* Front raises
* Rear delt flyes
* Upright rows

Arms:
* Bicep curls (dumbbell or barbell)
* Tricep dips
* Skull crushers
* Hammer curls
* Close-grip bench press

Core:

- Planks
- Russian twists
- Leg raises
- Bicycle crunches
- Swiss ball crunches

Cardio:
- Running
- Cycling
- Swimming
- HIIT workouts
- Rowing

Chapter 8: Understanding Cutting and Bulking for Fitness Success

When it comes to fitness and body composition goals, two terms that are often used are "cutting" and "bulking". These are distinct phases that individuals may go through to achieve specific objectives, whether it's losing body fat or building muscle mass. Understanding the difference between cutting and bulking can help you develop a targeted approach to optimize your fitness journey.

Cutting: Shedding Body Fat for a Lean Physique

Cutting, also known as a "cut" or "cutting phase", refers to a deliberate period during which you focus on reducing body fat while preserving muscle mass. The primary goal of cutting is to achieve a leaner and more defined physique. This is typically done by creating a caloric deficit, which means you consume fewer calories than you burn.

During a cutting phase, you may engage in activities such as cardiovascular exercise, resistance training, and a controlled diet to promote fat loss. Cardiovascular exercise helps burn calories and improve cardiovascular fitness, while resistance training helps maintain muscle mass and strength. A controlled diet involves monitoring your caloric intake, reducing processed foods, and prioritizing nutrient-dense foods.

<u>Bulking: Building Muscle Mass for Size and Strength</u>

Bulking, on the other hand, is a phase where the focus is on building muscle mass and increasing overall body size and strength. This typically involves consuming a caloric surplus, which means you consume more calories than you burn, to provide the extra energy needed for muscle growth.

During a bulking phase, you may engage in resistance training with progressively heavier weights to stimulate muscle hypertrophy or muscle growth. You may also increase your protein intake to support muscle repair and growth, along with sufficient carbohydrates and healthy fats for energy.

Key Differences between Cutting and Bulking

1. Caloric Intake: Cutting involves creating a caloric deficit, while bulking involves creating a caloric surplus.
2. Exercise Focus: Cutting may prioritize cardiovascular exercise to burn calories and promote fat loss while bulking may focus on resistance training to stimulate muscle growth.
3. Nutrient Intake: Cutting may prioritize nutrient-dense foods and portion control to manage caloric intake while bulking may prioritize higher protein intake for muscle growth and recovery.
4. Goal: The primary goal of cutting is to reduce body fat and achieve a leaner physique, while the primary goal of bulking is to build muscle mass and increase size and strength.
5. Timeframe: Cutting and bulking phases can vary in duration depending on individual goals and preferences.

Some people may cycle between cutting and bulking phases, while others may focus on one phase for an extended period.

Conclusion

Understanding the difference between cutting and bulking is crucial for tailoring your fitness approach to your specific goals. Whether you're aiming to reduce body fat or build muscle mass, having a clear understanding of these concepts can help you develop a strategic plan for your fitness journey. Remember to consult with a qualified fitness professional or nutritionist for personalized guidance and recommendations based on your individual needs and goals. With the right approach, you can optimize your fitness progress and achieve the results you desire.

Mastering the Cutting Phase: Shedding Body Fat for a Lean Physique

Cutting, also known as a "cut" or "cutting phase", is a crucial part of many fitness journeys, especially for those who are looking to reduce body fat and achieve a leaner, more defined physique. It requires a disciplined approach to create a caloric deficit, increase physical activity, and make strategic dietary choices. In this chapter, we will delve into the key principles and strategies to master the cutting phase and achieve your desired results.

Understanding the Importance of a Caloric Deficit

The cornerstone of a successful cutting phase is creating a caloric deficit, which means you consume fewer calories than you burn. This forces your body to tap into stored fat for energy, leading to fat loss over time. To create a caloric deficit, you can use a combination of decreasing your food intake and increasing your physical activity level.

Tracking and Managing Your Caloric Intake

One of the key aspects of cutting is to carefully monitor and manage your caloric intake. This involves understanding the macronutrient and micronutrient content of the foods you consume and tracking your daily caloric intake to ensure you're in a deficit. You can use a food tracking app or a food journal to keep track of your meals, snacks, and beverages, and calculate the total calories consumed.

Emphasizing Nutrient-Dense Foods

While reducing calories is important during cutting, it's equally important to prioritize nutrient-dense foods to ensure you're meeting your body's nutritional needs. Nutrient-dense foods are those that are rich in essential nutrients, such as vitamins, minerals, fibre, and protein while being relatively low in calories. Examples of nutrient-dense foods include lean proteins, whole grains, fruits, vegetables, and healthy fats. These foods can help you feel fuller for longer, provide the necessary nutrients for your body's functions, and support your workouts and recovery.

Increasing Physical Activity

To create a caloric deficit during cutting, you'll need to increase your physical activity level. This can involve a combination of cardiovascular exercise and resistance training. Cardiovascular exercise, such as running, cycling, or swimming, can help you burn calories and improve your cardiovascular fitness. Resistance training, such as weight lifting or bodyweight exercises, can help you maintain muscle mass and strength while losing fat. Aim for a well-rounded exercise routine that includes both cardiovascular and resistance training for optimal results.

Managing Hunger and Cravings

Cutting can sometimes be challenging as you may experience increased hunger and cravings due to the caloric deficit. To manage hunger, focus on consuming high-fibre foods that can help you feel fuller for longer, and drink plenty of water throughout the day. It's also important to be mindful of emotional eating and find alternative ways to cope with stress or other triggers. Planning and prepping your meals in advance can also help you make healthier choices and avoid giving in to cravings.

Prioritizing Rest and Recovery

Rest and recovery are equally important during the cutting phase as they are during any other phase of your fitness journey. Cutting requires a disciplined approach to diet and exercise, and it's important to give your body the time it needs to recover and repair. Make sure to get adequate sleep, prioritize rest days in your exercise routine, and listen to your body's signals to avoid overtraining or injuries.

Staying Consistent and Patient

Cutting can be a challenging phase as it requires consistent effort and patience. Results may not happen overnight, and it's important to stay committed to your plan and be patient with the process. Avoid drastic or unsustainable measures that promise quick results, and instead focus on creating healthy and sustainable habits that you can maintain in the long term.

<u>Incorporating Flexibility and Mindfulness</u>

Lastly, it is important to incorporate flexibility and mindfulness into your cutting phase. Being flexible with your approach allows you to adapt to different situations, such as social events or unexpected changes in your routine, without feeling deprived or overwhelmed. It's okay to indulge in a treat or enjoy a special occasion, as long as you are mindful of your choices and make efforts to balance them out with healthier options and increased physical activity.

Practicing mindfulness can also help you become more aware of your body's hunger and fullness cues, as well as your emotions and triggers for emotional eating. Mindful eating involves paying attention to your food, eating slowly, and savouring each bite. This can help you develop a healthier relationship with food and avoid mindless eating, which can easily derail your cutting goals.

Here's a 7-day workout routine focused on cutting, which is designed to help you burn fat, maintain muscle mass, and improve your overall fitness:

Day 1: Full-Body Resistance Training

- Warm-up: 5-10 minutes of light cardiovascular exercise (e.g., brisk walking, cycling, or rowing)

- Resistance Training: Perform compound exercises targeting major muscle groups such as squats, deadlifts, bench presses, rows, and overhead presses. Aim for 3-4 sets of 8-12 reps with challenging weights.
- Cardiovascular Exercise: Finish with 20-30 minutes of moderate-intensity cardio (e.g., running, cycling, or elliptical).

Day 2: Rest Day or Active Recovery

- Take a rest day or engage in low-intensity activities such as yoga, stretching, or light walking to promote recovery and reduce muscle soreness.

Day 3: High-Intensity Interval Training (HIIT)

- Warm-up: 5-10 minutes of dynamic stretching and mobility exercises
- HIIT Workout: Alternate between high-intensity exercises (e.g., sprints, burpees, or jump squats) and brief periods of rest. Aim for 10-15 minutes of intense work, followed by a cool-down and stretching.

Day 4: Upper Body Resistance Training

- Warm-up: 5-10 minutes of light cardiovascular exercise
- Resistance Training: Focus on upper body exercises such as pull-ups, push-ups, dumbbell curls, triceps dips, and lateral raises. Aim for 3-4 sets of 8-12 reps with challenging weights.
- Cardiovascular Exercise: Finish with 20-30 minutes of moderate-intensity cardio.

Day 5: Rest Day or Active Recovery

- Take another rest day or engage in low-intensity activities such as yoga, stretching, or light walking to promote recovery and reduce muscle soreness.

Day 6: Cardiovascular Endurance Training

- Warm-up: 5-10 minutes of light cardiovascular exercise
- Cardiovascular Exercise: Engage in sustained aerobic exercise such as running, cycling, swimming, or rowing for 30-45 minutes at a moderate intensity.

Day 7: Total Body Circuit Training

- Warm-up: 5-10 minutes of dynamic stretching and mobility exercises
- Circuit Training: Create a circuit of resistance exercises targeting different muscle groups (e.g., squats, lunges, push-ups, rows, and planks) and perform them in succession with minimal rest. Aim for 3-4 sets of 10-15 reps with moderate weights.
- Cardiovascular Exercise: Finish with 20-30 minutes of moderate-intensity cardio.

Note: It's essential to adjust the weight, sets, and reps based on your fitness level and progression. It's also crucial to include proper nutrition, hydration, and adequate rest to support your cutting goals and promote recovery.

Always consult with a qualified fitness professional or healthcare provider before starting any exercise program, especially if you have any health concerns or medical conditions. It's important to listen to your body, progress gradually, and make adjustments as needed to ensure safety and effectiveness in your workout routine.

In conclusion, the cutting phase is a challenging but essential part of many fitness journeys. It requires creating a caloric deficit, increasing physical activity, and making strategic dietary choices. By tracking and managing your caloric intake, prioritizing nutrient-dense foods, increasing physical activity, managing hunger and cravings, prioritizing rest and recovery, staying consistent and patient, and incorporating flexibility and mindfulness, you can successfully navigate the cutting phase and achieve your desired results. Remember to always consult with a healthcare professional or a qualified nutritionist or dietitian before making any significant changes to your diet or exercise routine, and listen to your body's signals throughout the process. Stay committed, stay focused, and stay positive, knowing that your hard work and dedication will pay off in the end, helping you achieve a leaner, healthier, and more confident version of yourself.

Bulking Up - Building Lean Muscle Mass for Strength and Size

The bulking phase is a period of intentional weight gain to build lean muscle mass. It involves increasing your caloric intake, primarily through an increase in protein and carbohydrates, to provide your body with the energy and nutrients needed to support muscle growth. Here are some key principles and strategies to consider during the bulking phase:

1. **Calorie Surplus:** To support muscle growth, you need to consume more calories than your body burns. This means creating a calorie surplus by eating more calories than you burn through your daily activities and exercise. It's important to calculate your daily caloric needs based on your age, gender, weight, activity level, and fitness goals, and then aim to consume around 250-500 calories above your maintenance level to promote muscle growth.

2. **Protein Intake:** Protein is crucial for muscle repair and growth. Aim to consume a sufficient amount of protein with each meal and snack during your bulking phase. Good sources of protein include lean meats, poultry, fish, eggs, dairy products, legumes, nuts, and seeds. Aim to consume approximately 1.6-2.2 grams of protein per kilogram of body weight per day to support muscle growth.

3. **Carbohydrate Intake:** Carbohydrates are an important energy source during bulking, as they provide the fuel needed for intense workouts and help replenish glycogen stores in muscles. Choose complex carbohydrates such as whole grains, fruits, vegetables, and starchy vegetables for sustained energy throughout the day.

4. **Resistance Training:** Resistance training, such as weightlifting or bodyweight exercises, is essential for building lean muscle mass during the bulking phase. Focus on compound exercises that target multiple muscle groups, such as squats, deadlifts, bench presses, and rows, to stimulate maximum muscle growth. Gradually increase the weight and resistance over time to progressively challenge your muscles.

5. **Rest and Recovery:** Adequate rest and recovery are crucial for muscle growth. During the bulking phase, aim to get

enough sleep, usually 7-9 hours per night, to allow your muscles to repair and grow. Avoid overtraining and give yourself enough time to recover between workouts to prevent injury and optimize muscle growth.

6. Monitoring Progress: Keep track of your progress during the bulking phase by regularly measuring your body weight, body fat percentage, and muscle mass. Use this data to make adjustments to your caloric intake, macronutrient ratios, and exercise routine as needed to continue making progress toward your muscle-building goals.

7. Adjusting Macros: While protein and carbohydrates are important during bulking, don't neglect healthy fats. Fats are important for hormone production, joint health, and overall health. Include sources of healthy fats in your diet such as avocados, nuts, seeds, olive oil, and fatty fish like salmon.

8. Consistency: Building lean muscle mass takes time and consistency. Be patient and committed to your bulking phase, as results may not happen overnight. Stay consistent with your nutrition and exercise plan, and be prepared to put in the effort and dedication required to achieve your muscle-building goals.

9. Mindset: Maintaining a positive mindset is crucial during the bulking phase. Be prepared for changes in your body composition, such as an increase in body weight and some body fat, as this is a natural part of the bulking process. Embrace the progress you are making in terms of increased strength and muscle mass, and avoid negative self-talk or comparison to others.

In conclusion, the bulking phase is an essential part of building lean muscle mass for strength and size. It requires creating a calorie surplus, prioritizing protein and carbohydrates, engaging in regular resistance training, getting adequate rest and recovery, monitoring progress, adjusting macros, being consistent, and maintaining a positive mindset. By following these principles and strategies, you can optimize your bulking phase and make significant progress toward your muscle-building goals.

It's important to note that bulking is not an excuse to indulge in unhealthy eating habits or neglect cardiovascular exercise. It's still crucial to prioritize overall health and well-being by including a variety of nutrient-dense foods in your diet, staying hydrated, and engaging in regular cardiovascular exercise to support cardiovascular health and maintain overall fitness.

Remember, the goal of bulking is to build lean muscle mass, not just gain weight indiscriminately. It's important to focus on progressive resistance training and monitor your progress to ensure that the weight gained is primarily muscle mass, rather than excess body fat.

Furthermore, it's essential to listen to your body and make adjustments to your nutrition and exercise plan as needed. Everyone's body is unique, and what works for one person may not work for another. Pay attention to how your body responds to the bulking phase and make adjustments accordingly to optimize your results.

In summary, the bulking phase is a strategic approach to building lean muscle mass for strength and size. It requires a calorie surplus, sufficient protein and carbohydrate intake, resistance training, rest and recovery, progress monitoring, macro adjustments, consistency, and a positive mindset. By following these principles and strategies, you can effectively navigate the bulking phase and make significant progress toward your muscle-building goals. Remember to prioritize overall health and well-being, listen to your body, and make adjustments as needed for optimal results.

Here's a 7-day workout routine focused on bulking, which is designed to help you build muscle mass, increase strength, and improve your overall fitness:

Day 1: Chest and Triceps

- Warm-up: 5-10 minutes of light cardiovascular exercise
- Resistance Training: Perform compound exercises targeting the chest muscles such as bench press, incline bench press, and dips, along with triceps exercises like triceps dips, triceps extensions, and close-grip bench press. Aim for 3-4 sets of 8-12 reps with challenging weights.
- Cardiovascular Exercise: Optional, depending on your energy levels and goals.

Day 2: Back and Biceps

- Warm-up: 5-10 minutes of light cardiovascular exercise
- Resistance Training: Focus on compound exercises for the back muscles such as pull-ups, rows, and deadlifts, along with biceps exercises like curls and hammer curls. Aim for 3-4 sets of 8-12 reps with challenging weights.
- Cardiovascular Exercise: Optional, depending on your energy levels and goals.

Day 3: Rest Day or Active Recovery

- Take a rest day or engage in low-intensity activities such as yoga, stretching, or light walking to promote recovery and reduce muscle soreness.

Day 4: Legs and Shoulders

- Warm-up: 5-10 minutes of light cardiovascular exercise
- Resistance Training: Perform compound exercises targeting the leg muscles such as squats, lunges, and leg presses, along with shoulder exercises like shoulder presses, lateral raises, and front raises. Aim for 3-4 sets of 8-12 reps with challenging weights.
- Cardiovascular Exercise: Optional, depending on your energy levels and goals.

Day 5: Rest Day or Active Recovery

- Take another rest day or engage in low-intensity activities such as yoga, stretching, or light walking to promote recovery and reduce muscle soreness.

Day 6: Full-Body Resistance Training

- Warm-up: 5-10 minutes of light cardiovascular exercise
- Resistance Training: Perform compound exercises targeting major muscle groups such as squats, deadlifts, bench presses, rows, and overhead presses. Aim for 3-4 sets of 8-12 reps with challenging weights.
- Cardiovascular Exercise: Optional, depending on your energy levels and goals.

Day 7: Arms and Abs

- Warm-up: 5-10 minutes of light cardiovascular exercise
- Resistance Training: Focus on biceps, triceps, and abdominal exercises such as curls, extensions, skull crushers, cable crunches, and leg raises. Aim for 3-4 sets of 8-12 reps with challenging weights.
- Cardiovascular Exercise: Optional, depending on your energy levels and goals.

Note: It's essential to adjust the weight, sets, and reps based on your fitness level and progression. It's also crucial to include proper nutrition, hydration, and adequate rest to support your bulking goals and promote recovery.

Always consult with a qualified fitness professional or healthcare provider before starting any exercise program, especially if you have any health concerns or medical conditions. It's important to listen to your body, progress gradually, and make adjustments as needed to ensure safety and effectiveness in your workout routine.

A STRONG

BODY

IS A

STRONG

MIND

www.ingramcontent.com/pod-product-compliance
Lightning Source LLC
Chambersburg PA
CBHW050053260726
48658CB00005B/1918